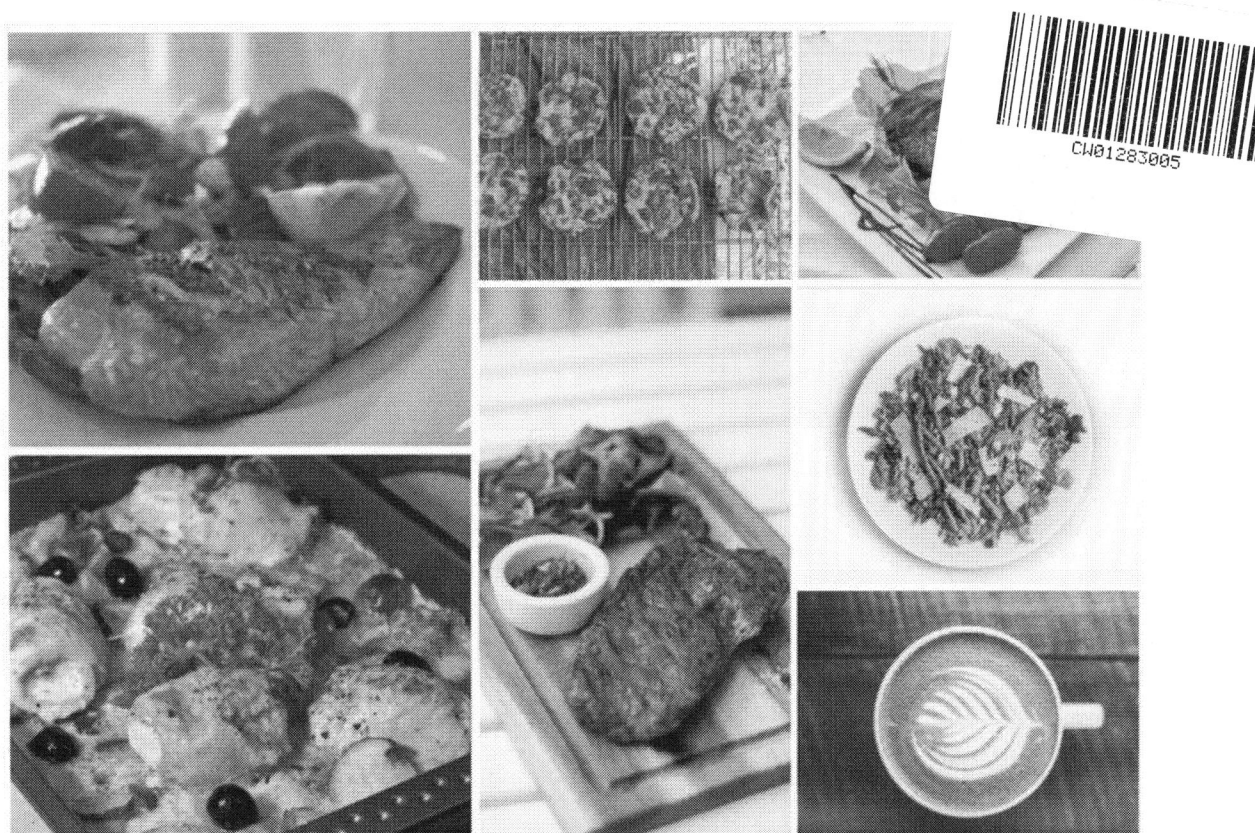

KETO AFTER 50
BEST SECRETS TO BURN FAT

NEW KETO DIET AND WEIGHT LOSS 18 POUNDS IN 4 DAYS MEAL PLAN

MALINA PRONTO

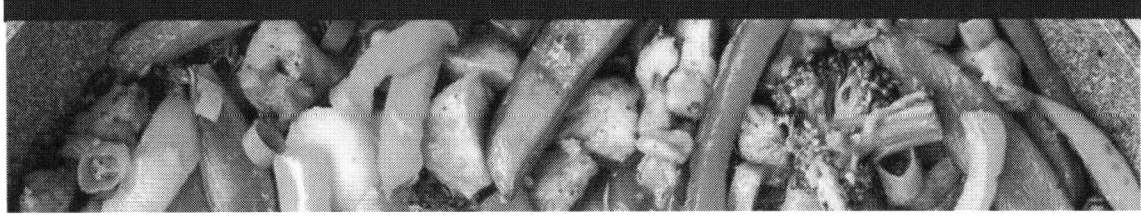

Keto After 50: Best Secrets To Burn Fat: New Keto Diet And Weight Loss | 18 Pounds In 4 Days Meal Plan

Introduction

A ketogenic diet is basically an eating regimen that changes over your body from consuming sugar to consuming fat. Around 99% of the wold's populace has an eating routine that makes their body consume sugar.

Subsequently, starches are their essential fuel source utilized in the wake of processing carbs. This procedure makes individuals put on weight, in any case, an eating regimen of fat and ketones will cause weight reduction. As you ask what are you ready to eat a ketogenic diet, as a matter of first importance, eat up to 30 to 50 grams of carbs every day.

Next, permit us to find more about what you'll wear your plate and the way the ketogenic diet influences your wellbeing.

Learn The Secrets To Burn Fat

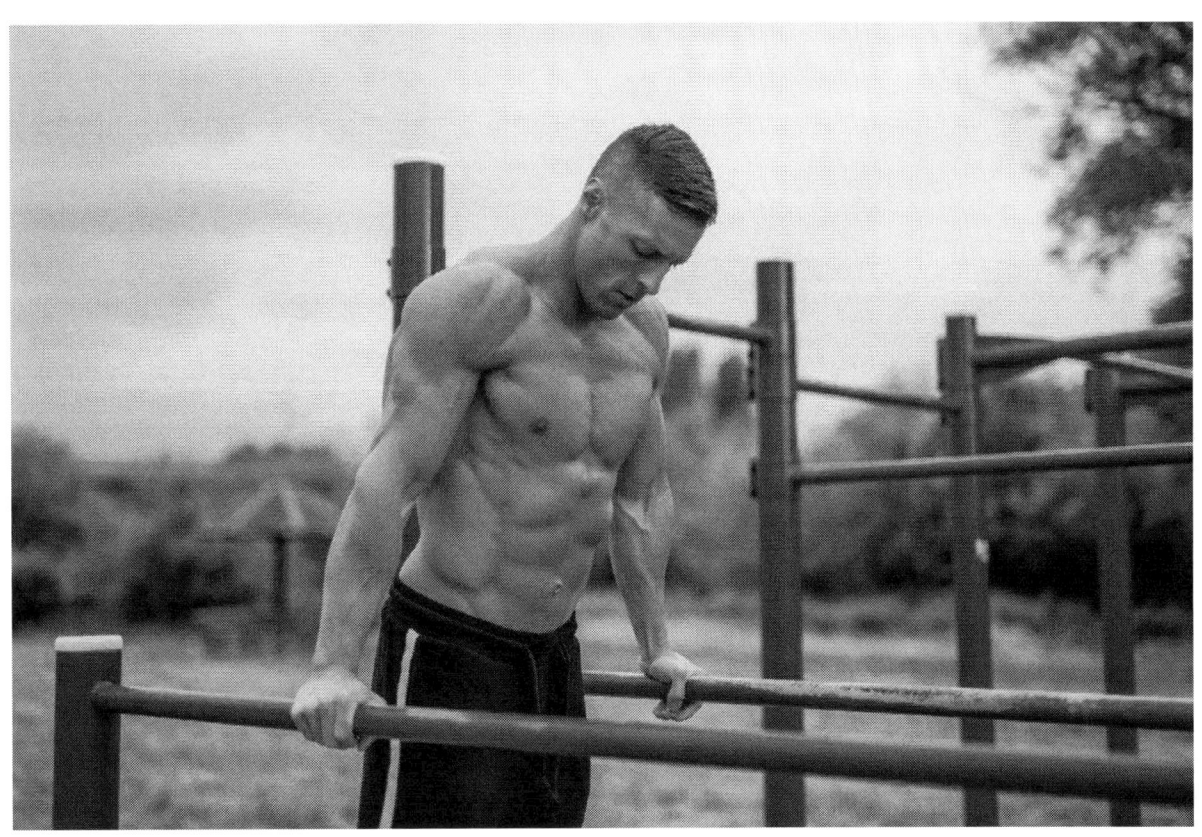

The Importance Of Sugar Precaution On The Ketogenic Diet

Keto shifts your body from a sugar burner to a fat burner by eliminating the dietary sugar derived from carbohydrates. the primary obvious reduction you ought to make from your current diet is sugar and sugary foods. Although sugar may be a definite target for deletion, the ketogenic diet focuses on the limitation of carbohydrates.

we'd like to observe out for sugar during a number of various sorts of foods and nutrients. Even a white potato which is carb-heavy might not taste sweet to your tongue like sugar.

But once it hits your bloodstream after digestion, those carbs add the straightforward sugar referred to as glucose to your body. the reality is, our body can only store such a lot of glucose before it dumps it elsewhere in our system. Excess glucose becomes what's referred to as the fat which accumulates in our stomach region, love handles, etc.

Protein And It's Place In Keto

One source of carbohydrates that some people overlook in their diet is protein. Overconsumption of protein consistent with the tolerance level of your body will end in weight gain. Because our body converts excess protein into sugar, we must moderate the quantity of protein we eat. Moderation of our protein intake is a component of the way to eat ketogenic and reduce. First of all, identify your own tolerance of daily protein and use it as a guide to take care of the optimal intake of the nutrient. Second, choose your protein from foods like organic cage-free eggs and grass-fed meats. Finally, create meals in variety that are delicious and maintain your interest within the diet.

as an example, a 5-ounce steak and a couple of eggs can provide a perfect amount of daily protein for a few people.

Caloric Intake On The Ketogenic Diet

Calories are another important consideration for what are you able to eat a ketogenic diet. Energy derived from the calories within the food we consume helps our body to stay functional. Hence, we must eat enough calories so as to satisfy our daily nutritional requirements. Counting calories may be a burden for several people that are on other diets.

But as a ketogenic dieter, you do not need to worry nearly the maximum amount about calorie counting. most of the people on a low-carb diet remain satisfied by eating a daily amount of 1500-1700 kcals in calories.

Fats, the great & The Bad

Fat isn't bad, actually many good healthy fats exist in whole foods like nuts, seeds, and vegetable oil. Healthy fats are an integral part of the ketogenic diet and are available as spreads, snacks, and toppings.

Misconceptions with regard to eating fat are that a high amount of it's unhealthy and causes weight gain. While both statements are during a sense true, the fat which we consume isn't the direct explanation for the fat which appears on our body. Rather, the sugar from each nutrient we consume is what eventually becomes the fat on our body.

Balance Your Nutrients Wisely

Digestion causes the sugars we eat to soak up into the bloodstream and therefore the excess amount transfer into our fat cells.

High carbohydrate and high protein eating will end in excess body fat because there's sugar content in these nutrients. So excessive eating of any nutrient is unhealthy and causes weight gain. But a healthy diet consists of a balance of protein, carbohydrates, and fats consistent with the tolerance levels of your body.

Just about everyone can accomplish a ketogenic diet with enough persistence and energy. additionally, we will moderate a variety of bodily conditions naturally with keto. Insulin resistance, elevated blood glucose, inflammation, obesity, type-2 diabetes are some health conditions that keto can help to stabilize.

Each of those unhealthy conditions will reduce and normalize for the victim who follows a healthy ketogenic diet. Low-carb, high-fat and moderate protein whole foods provide the life-changing health benefits of this diet.

The Keto Diet and Weight Loss

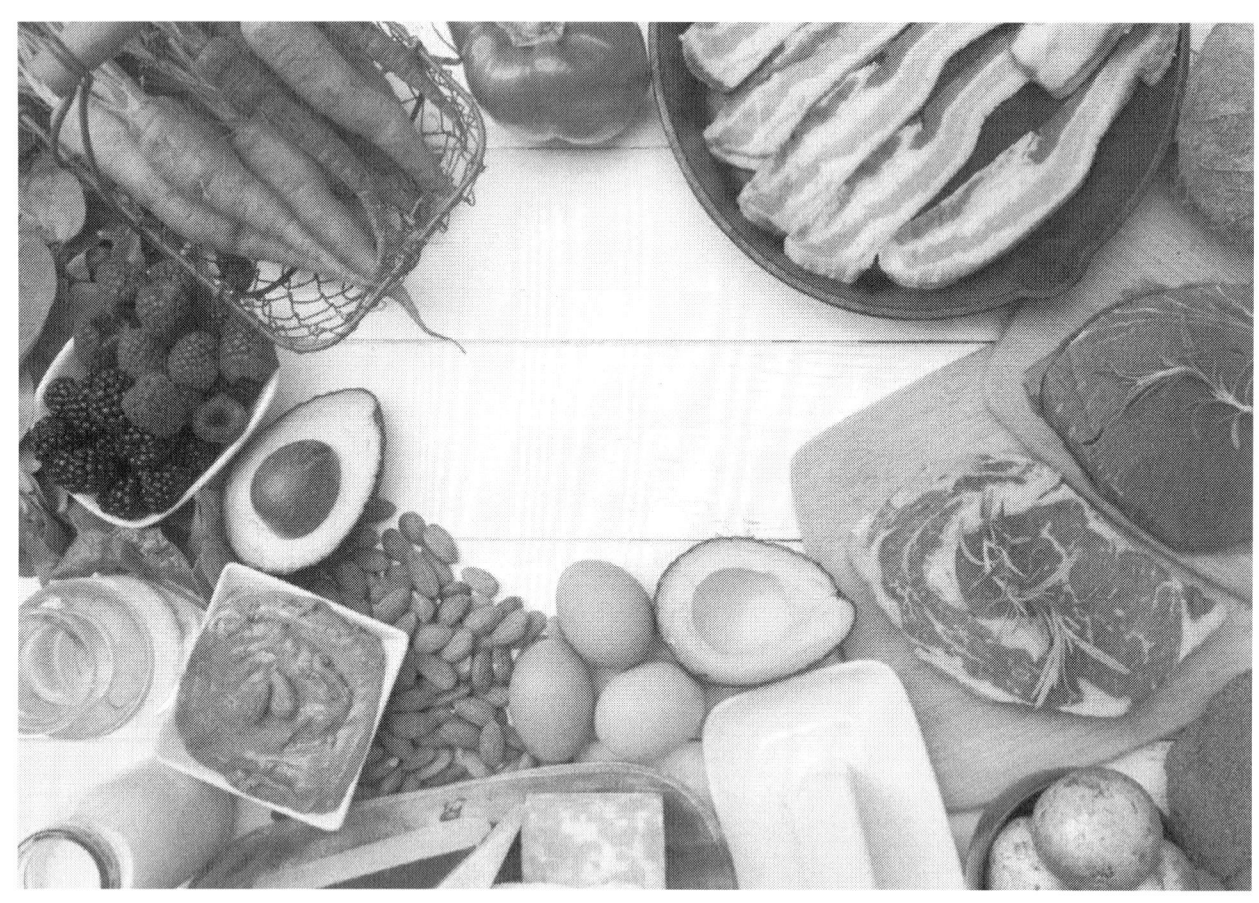

If you've got had a desire to shed some extra pounds, then perhaps you'll have encountered a ketogenic diet, which is popularly referred to as Keto diet. it's a well-liked weight loss plan that promises significant weight loss during a short time.

But faraway from what most of the people believe it to be, the diet isn't a magical tool for weight loss. a bit like the other diet, it takes time, requires tons of adjustment and tracking to ascertain results.

What is the Keto diet?

The keto diet is aimed at putting your body in Ketosis. This diet plan is typically low carb with a high intake of healthy fats, vegetables, and sufficient proteins. within this diet, there's also a stress on avoiding highly processed foods and sugars.

There are several sorts of Keto diets: standard ketogenic, cyclical, targeted, and therefore the high-protein diets. The difference in them depends on the carb intake. the quality ketogenic diet is low carb, high fat and adequate protein is that the most recommended.

Is the Keto Diet Safe?

Most critics of the Keto diet say that it's not safe due to the stress on consuming high-fat content. this is often guided by the misunderstanding that fats are bad for you. On the contrary, healthy fats are literally excellent for you.

With this diet, you get many fats from healthy sources like avocado, nuts, fish, butter, eggs, copra oil, palm oil, seeds like chia, and meat.

How Does the Keto Diet Aid in Weight Loss?

So how does the keto diet really work and help your body lose excess pounds? When on a high carb diet, your body uses glucose from carbohydrates and sugars to fuel body activities. When on a ketogenic diet, you supply the body with minimal amounts of carbs and sugars.

With reduced sugar and carbs supply, the glucose levels within the body are depleted causing the body to seem for energy sources. The body, therefore, turns to stored fats for energy which is why the Keto diet results in weight loss.

This condition where your body burns fats for energy aside from carbs is named ketosis. When your body goes into ketosis, it produced ketones because of the fuel source instead of counting on glucose. Ketones and glucose are the sole two power sources that fuel the brain.

Benefits of Ketosis and therefore the Keto diet

Besides just aiding in weight loss, putting the body in ketosis comes with other health benefits too. Here are a number of them:

Enhanced mental clarity

Improved physical energy

Steady blood glucose levels which make it an honest remedy for epilepsy and diabetes

Improved and enhanced skin tones

Lower cholesterol levels

Hormone regulation especially in women

The Ketogenic diet is one of the simplest diets you'll follow for weight loss and to reinforce your overall health. The diet also can be used for youngsters who are overweight.

There are numerous studies that support the diet showing significant results especially when including exe

Is an expert author on matters to try to to with weight loss.

18 Pounds in 4 Days Meal Plan

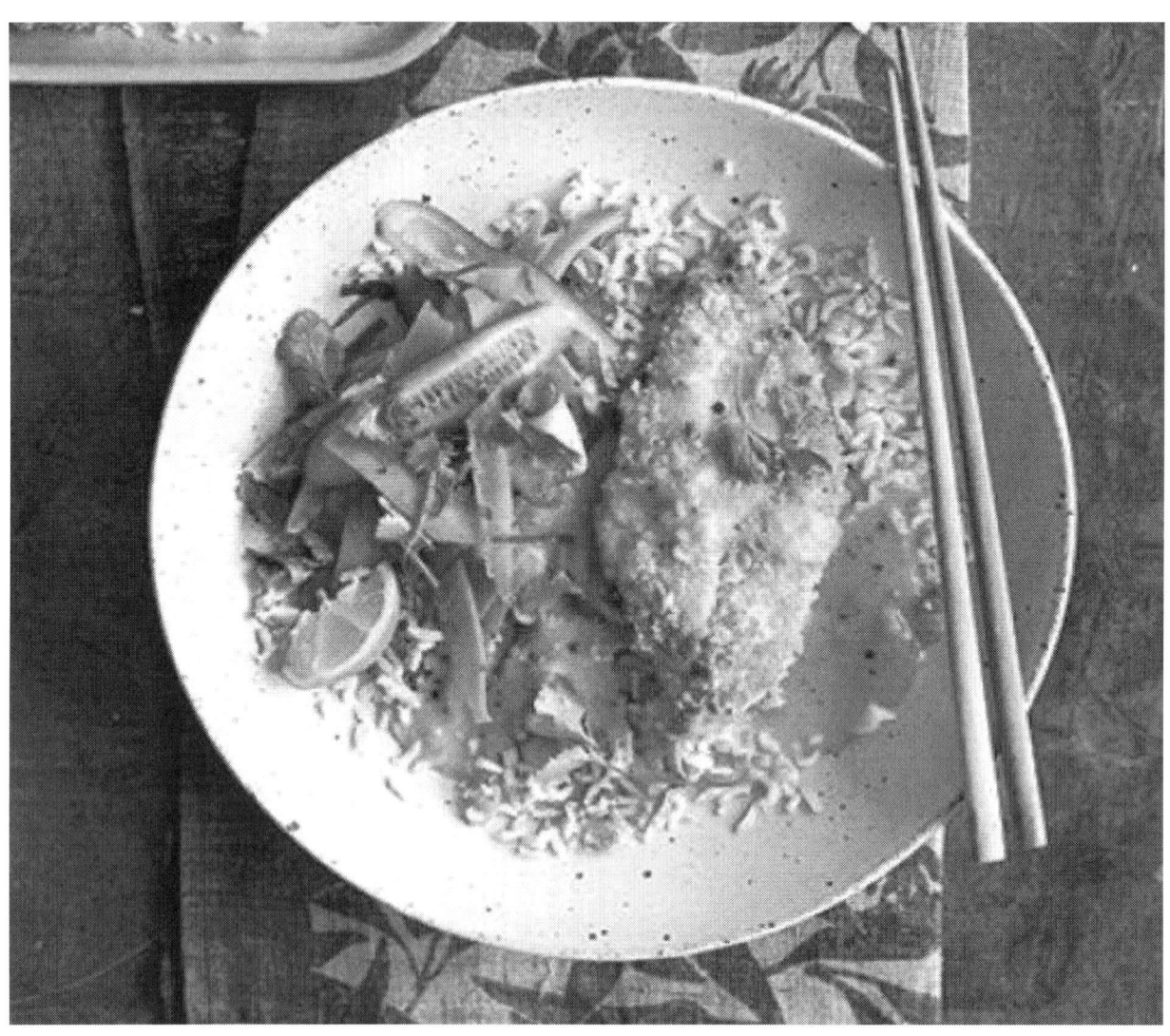

One of the foremost controversial weight loss programs online today is that the Lose 18 Pounds in 4 Days hotel plan program, created by James Zeta. It's one among those programs that nobody knows an excessive amount of about but it still creates an excellent deal of interest.

So, what's this hotel plan, and does it really work? are you able to really lose18 lbs in 4 days?

There are testimonials on the official site of this program which state that you simply can and that I can't argue with them, so I assume that it's possible.

However, this is often a rather extreme weight loss which can not be that good for people that want future results.

The way this program work is thru a really low calorie and strict eating plan. For 4 days, you always eat eggs, vegetables, and a touch fruit. Don't expect high quantities of food. you continue to got to drop tons of weight in a particularly short period of your time. However, since you eat so little for just 4 days, it isn't something regrettable. you'll roll in the hay.

You do get an in-depth eating plan during this program which may be a major advantage.

However, some experts believe that this type of ultra-fast weight loss are often bad for your health as it's sort of a blast wave to your body. additionally, fast weight loss can cause metabolic slowdown which suggests that your metabolism slows down which makes it harder for you to continue losing weight within the end of the day or to take care of it far into the longer term.

If you've got an occasion arising and wish to lose tons of weight fast, the 18 lbs in 4 days plan may go for you. If you've got a touch longer to reduce , it might probably be better to settle on a more gradual program.

Why Did I Choose a Ketogenic Lifestyle

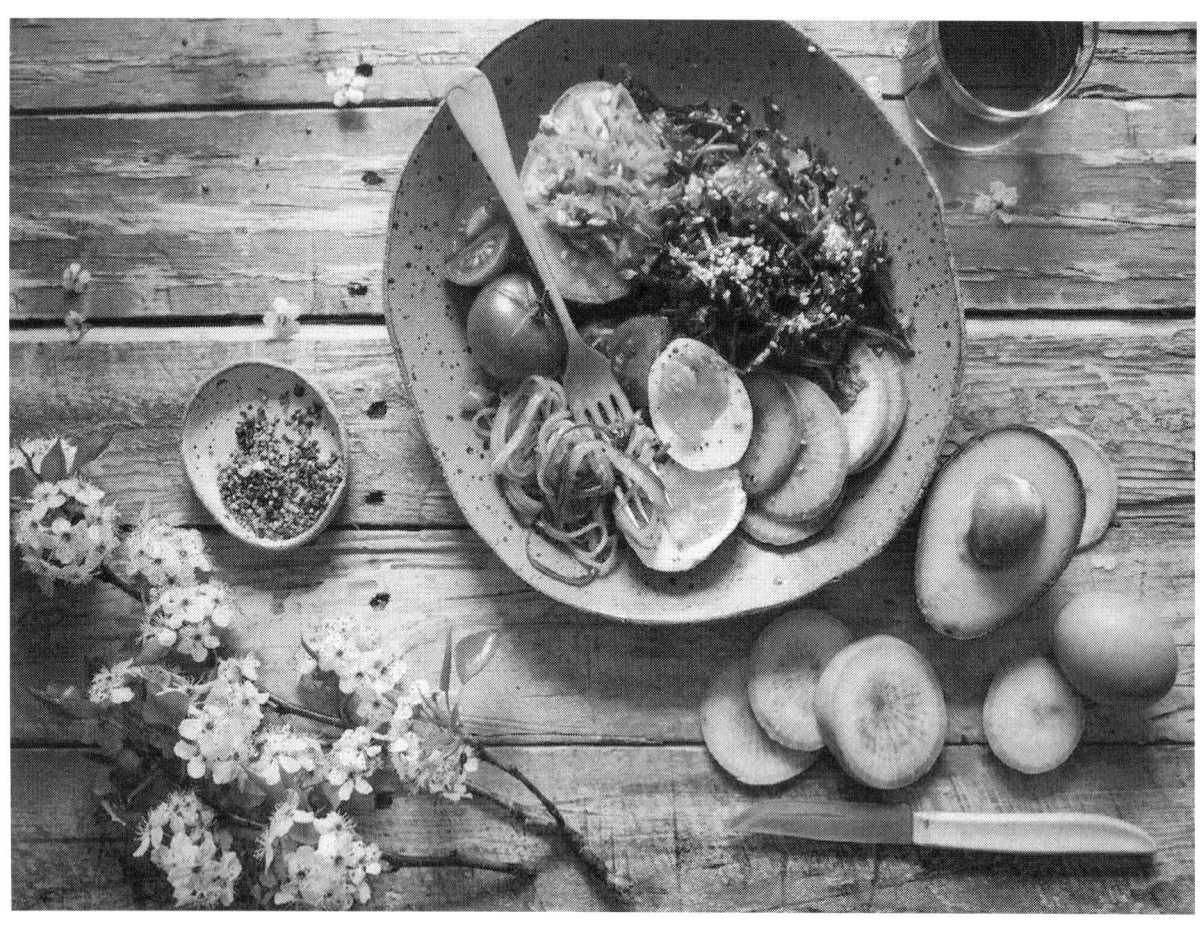

Initially, once I first started examining ketogenic eating, my primary goal ended up being to shed extra pounds. I'm what I call a "recovering fatass", in just an equivalent way that somebody who has quit drinking could all right be referred to as a "recovering alcoholic". I've struggled with my weight all my life, and that I fully expect that albeit I'm ready to accomplish the goals I've selected (and I will), the struggle won't be over. I feel this is often a crucial realization for anyone trying to reduce to possess, but that's a topic for an additional day.

The first thing that drew me into a ketogenic diet as how to reduce was any time you strictly limit your carbohydrate intake, you will be ready to force (I'm keen on saying "train") your system to settle on fat as fuel as against counting on carbs. I'm curious about life-hacking and "mind over matter", and therefore the simple incontrovertible fact that I'd be taking additional control of my body became an enormous incentive.

On top of the premise that I could train my body to use fat as fuel, I additionally was interested in the claims of reduced hunger and appetite. As anyone who has ever experimented with diet before knows, the hunger pangs are usually awful to manage, and whenever willpower slips at the incorrect time it isn't hard to urge obviate every week's worth of careful eating with one binge. many of us generally state that after a limited time eating a ketogenic diet (2-4 weeks for most) they find they're often just not as hungry as they were before, even on a calorie-reduced diet! Not being as hungry means fewer chances to ruin on a diet plan, which may be a major plus to me.

Finally, I found myself fascinated with the food I might manage to eat and keep my ketogenic diet. I've for ages been interested in food beyond just eating and thus I enjoy cooking an excellent deal, of course, if you'll find one main truth to food, it really is that fat equals flavor! to return across a diet program that only allowed, but encouraged, fat as the food was like discovering the last word goal. However, as I've told anyone I've discussed ketogenic eating with, it isn't a diet plan that means you'll eat whatever you fancy in whatever quantities you would like.

Losing weight is, in essence, math... if you dine in fewer calories than you expend, you'll expect to drop weight, full stop. But by making the calories I'm taking in delicious,

I won't crave extras, and I am getting to be more likely to follow my plan. Or at the smallest amount, this is often the idea.

So there you've got it. this is often just a fast guide to a couple of the items that drew me to ketogenic eating, we'll touch on the precise science behind this diet on another day. a minimum of immediately you recognize what got me moving on my fat-burning journey!

Is Your Goal Really Weight Loss and Diet

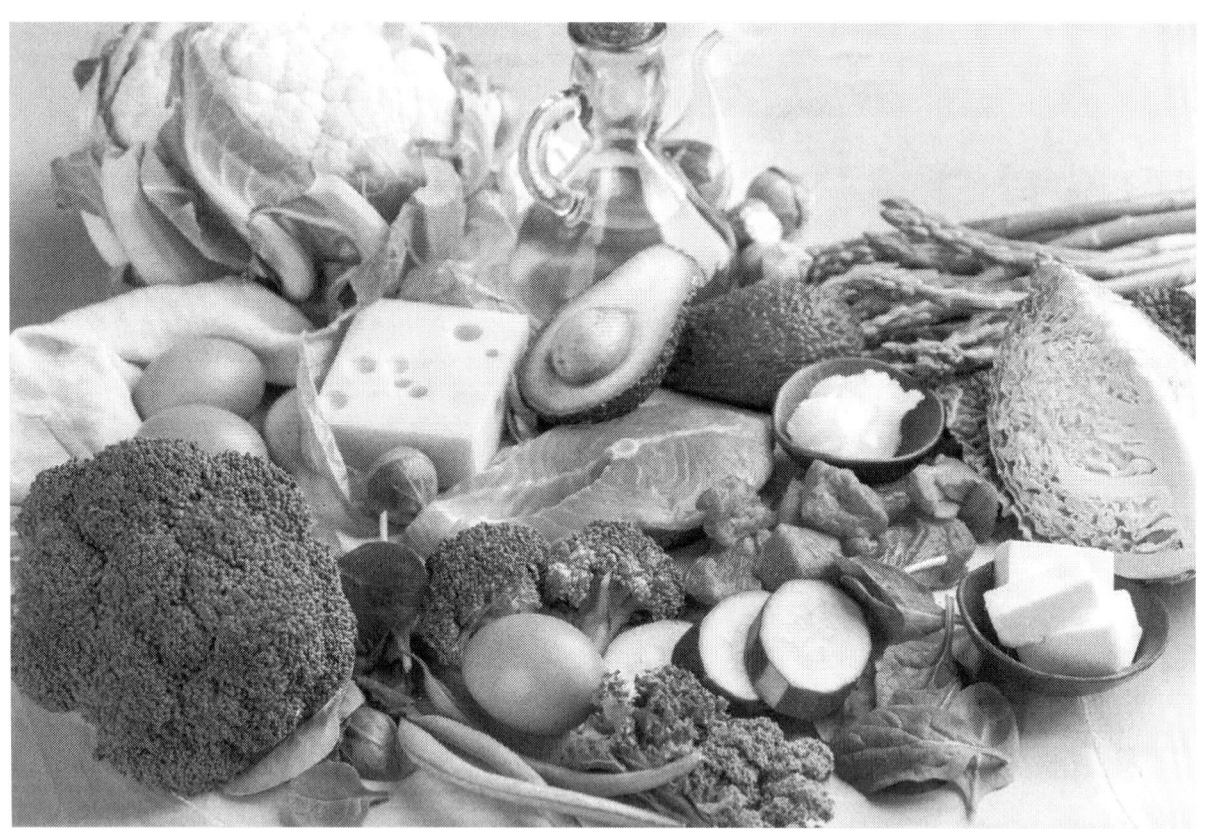

Are you ashamed of your weight? does one have a goal weight that you simply want to succeed in through weight loss? I'd say so, it has been pushed into our brains repeatedly over and once again that "weight loss" is what we would like to accomplish. There are weight loss guides, weight loss supplements, and lots of other things that push "weight loss". many of us even set their goals to be at a particular weight. Additionally, the medical profession has developed an "ideal weight" chart, which may further increase the confusion about weight loss.

Now, let me ask you an issue.

Is your goal really weight loss?

Unless you're trying to form a weight class for wrestling or another sport with weight classes, you'll think that your goal is weight loss, but it really isn't. you're trying to lose that flubber stuff attached to your body called FAT. Correct?

So then, why can we measure our progress by what proportion we weigh? Why can we tread on the toilet scale and hope that those numbers are going to be less than before? You see, our weight is suffering from quite just what proportion fat is on our body. other factors include water, muscle, glycogen, and clearly, if we've eaten anything earlier or used the toilet lately.

Our water weight fluctuates constantly. as an example, once we exhale water vapor comes out. once we sweat, we are sweating out water. There also are more factors which will affect the quantity of water in our body. Water is what usually causes those random gains or losses of a pound or two in weight which will cause you to happy or sad. it's almost physiologically impossible to lose a pound of fat in at some point.

One reason the low-carb or no-carb (also called ketogenic) diets are so attractive is due to the massive initial loss of weight. However, this weight isn't necessarily fat.

When carbohydrates are restricted the body features a backup store of them located within the liver and muscles within the sort of something called glycogen. The physical body can store approximately 400 grams of glycogen. In larger individuals, this number can increase. additionally to the present, for every gram of glycogen stored within the physical body, 3 grams of water also are stored. If you work it out, this is able to equate to about 1600 grams (3.5 pounds) of glycogen and water.

When you stop or limit your consumption of carbohydrates, your body starts using its glycogen stores.

After a few days that 1600 grams (3.5 pounds) of glycogen and water are gone. Also, as an adaptation to the restriction of carbohydrates, your body produces this stuff called ketones. Ketones also appear to possess a diuretic effect, which might mean a good greater loss of water.

In addition to water, if you've got been understanding lately to hurry along with your "weight loss" (you mean fat loss, right?) progress you almost certainly have gained some muscle doing so. This gain in muscle also can affect the numbers you see on the size. Muscle is additionally more dense than fat.

You may be wondering how you're getting to measure your progress now that the size doesn't suggest the maximum amount because it won't to. Well, there are several methods to live your body fat percentage. None of those methods are 100% accurate, but they're going to be far more useful than the utilization of a scale.

One of the only ways is to use a caliper. you'll usually find these at your local sporting goods/fitness shop. If you cannot find them locally, you'll get them organized off the web. Calipers measure the thickness of a skin fold on your triceps.

Then there are directions that accompany the caliper that show you ways to use the amount you get to derive your body rich person.

If you do not want to travel out and buy some calipers, there's a body rich person calculator on my website. The calculator uses the circumference of several parts of your body then plugs them into a formula developed by the U.S. Navy to derive an approximation of your body rich person.

There also are far more accurate ways to live your body rich people like buoyancy testing or the utilization of special lasers.

If you enforce knowing your progress by weight loss and need to use a scale, attempt to weigh yourself at an equivalent time every day. Probably the simplest time would be right once you awaken within the morning and before you are doing anything.

So, your new goal should be to draw a bead on fat loss and not weight loss. Don't necessarily trust the size all the time because it are often deceiving - your weight is suffering from quite just what proportion fat you've got gained or lost. additionally , it's almost physiologically impossible to realize or lose a pound of fat in at some point .

Losing Weight by Ketosis

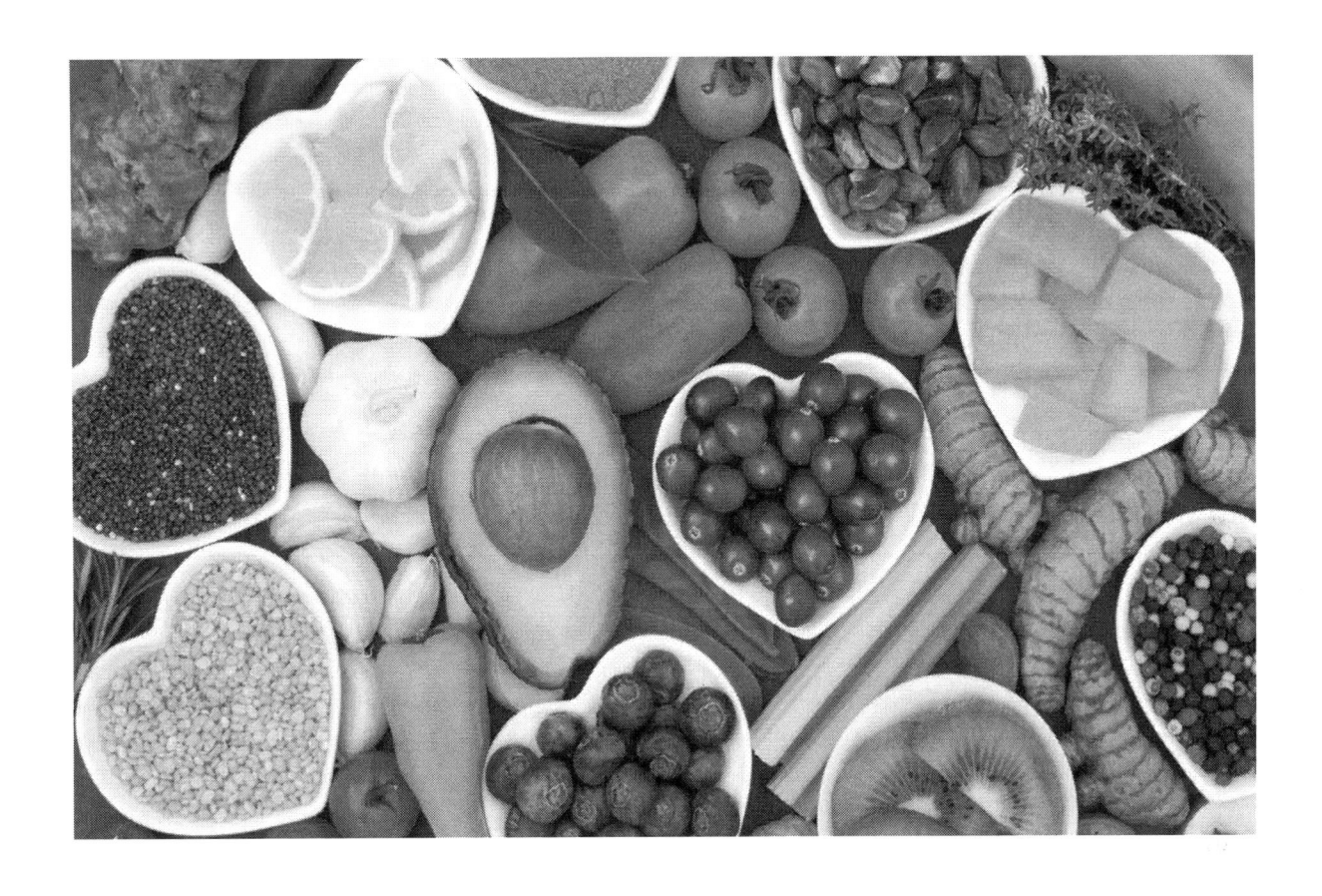

The process of burning fat from your body by reducing your carbohydrate intake is understood as losing weight by ketosis. within the past 10 years approximately we've heard mention of the Atkins diet which is predicated on the ketosis process.

A low carbohydrate diet uses ketosis or better said ketosis is how you experience weight loss from the low carbohydrate diet. The low-carbohydrate diet is nothing as compared to the reduced-calorie sort of diet, the 2 are completely different from the load loss from calorie reduction is from fat and lean muscle tissue whereas your metabolism is really slowing down which actually makes losing weight slower and harder and gaining weight back simpler.

Ketones are produced by the breakdown of fatty acids within the liver then which ends up in ketones being created. Ketones once created won't revert back to fat but are going to be excreted naturally from the body. This process is ketosis and is why the Atkins diet is carbohydrate restrictive, creating the ketosis process burns only fat and not muscle.

When there's an absence of sugar and glucose within the bloodstream your body will produce ketones for energy.

this is often what the Atkins diet is all about. When your body is creating ketones this is often referred to as ketosis. At the arrival of the Atkins diet, people were saying that following a ketogenic diet was harmful to your health when actually it's a wild when your body is creating ketones for energy because there's no sugar or glucose available.

The reason you're dieting is that there's an absence of exercise and activity in your lifestyle. Exercise isn't really instrumental within the ketosis process, I'm inserting this reminder here that no matter what your weight-loss objective is or what goals you would like to realize, you would like to possess an exercise regime. you ought to develop this regime as a part of a healthy lifestyle which can cause an extended and meaningful life.

Ketosis and therefore the Atkins diet is simply the straightforward process of reducing your carbohydrate intake. there's the Atkins guide (available in stores or the internet) which can assist you through the varied stages of weight loss by the Atkins Diet, beginning where you'll consume only a few carbohydrates, then working up to the upkeep level where you'll enjoy a wider sort of foods in your diet. this is often the ketosis process in losing weight.

is simply your every day quite a guy who is an online marketing investigator by which I mean I even have done an excellent number of things with regard with internet marketing.

MALINA PRONTO

Printed in Great Britain
by Amazon